The Mind Diet Cookbook 2024

Title:
The Mind Diet Cookbook 2024

Subtitle

Delicious Brain-Enhancing Recipes for Memory, Focus, and Mental Clarity

ISBN: 9798862199963

TABLE OF CONTENT

INTRODUCTION

Welcome to The Mind Diet Cookbook 2024!

out on a journey to experience the flavors of a healthier brain, nurture your mind, and improve your cognitive fitness. We update the recipes and nutritional advice in this edition to help you use the Mind Diet to improve your brain health.

Discover the vital nutrients for a healthy brain, discover how to seamlessly apply Mind Diet principles to your daily life, and join us as we examine the intriguing science behind the Mind Diet.

You'll find a tempting selection of meals in this cookbook that are intended to improve your cognitive energy and mental clarity. Every dish is created with the health of your brain in mind, from filling breakfasts to healthy lunches, robust dinners, and delectable Set snacks.

Additionally, we'll show you how to throw brain-healthy get-togethers, modify the Mind Diet for special events, and develop mindful eating routines for get-togethers.

We've provided weekly meal plans and grocery lists to make your trip even more convenient, guaranteeing that you can effortlessly adopt the Mind Diet way of life. You'll discover useful advice on how to manage your stress, get in shape, practice mindfulness, and get enough sleep to keep your mind in good shape.

Therefore, "Mind Diet Cookbook 2024" is here to help you every step of the way, whether you're trying to make a lifestyle shift or want to improve your cognitive wellbeing. Join us in recognizing your dedication to bettering brain health and enjoy the tantalizing flavors of a more promising future.

Let's begin this culinary adventure with a more wholesome, contented mind!

Understanding the Mind Diet: A Path to Cognitive Wellness

We explore the core of the Mind Diet, a dietary strategy with scientific support that provides a revolutionary route to cognitive wellbeing, in the pages that follow. This chapter acts as your compass, directing you through the fundamental ideas and information that support the Mind Diet's capacity to hydrate and improve your brain.

Unlock the potential for increased cognitive function, a sharper memory, and mental clarity by learning the fascinating research that connects your dietary choices to brain health. We'll go through the essential vitamins, phytochemicals, and foods that have been proven to boost brain health so you can choose your meals wisely.

You will learn more about how the Mind Diet works to lower the risk of cognitive decline and neurodegenerative disorders throughout this chapter. The Mind Diet offers a holistic approach that emphasizes delicious, brain-boosting foods, whether you're looking for strategies to improve cognitive function as you age or are taking preventative measures to safeguard your brain.

Armed with the information and comprehension of the Mind Diet, you'll be prepared to make decisions that not only fuel your body but also improve your mental well-being as you set out on this culinary trip. This chapter is your road map to a healthier, sharper mind because the Mind Diet is more than simply a diet; it's a lifestyle that supports cognitive vibrancy.

So, let's get started by learning the Mind Diet's secrets and opening the door to a better, more exciting future for your cognitive fitness.

How This Cookbook Can Transform Your Brain Health

Welcome to a culinary journey that can improve your cognitive health and change the way your brain functions. This chapter examines the amazing ways that "Mind Diet Cookbook 2024" can be your dependable ally as you travel toward a healthier, happier mind.

1. **Inspiring Brain-Boosting Recipes:** Our collection of dishes has been painstakingly created to satisfy your palate while also giving your brain the vital nutrients it needs. Each dish is created to nourish your mind and assist you in realizing all its potential.

2. **Scientifically Informed Choices:** Our cookbook is based on the most recent academic studies on diet and mental health. You may choose foods that enhance your cognitive wellness with ease because we have simplified complex research discoveries into usable suggestions.

3. **Accessibility and Ease:** Our recipes are created to be accessible and simple to follow, regardless of whether you are a seasoned cook or a kitchen novice. To prepare meals that will make you feel more intellectually agile, you don't need to be a culinary genius.

4. **Meal Planning Made Simple:** To make your journey easier, we've supplied grocery lists and meal ideas. We've taken care of the planning so you don't have to worry about it and can focus on staying on the Mind Diet.

5. **Holistic Approach:** We investigate the broader facets of brain health in addition to recipes. You'll find advice on how to deal with stress, include exercise in your schedule, practice mindfulness, and place a high priority on getting enough sleep—all things that support cognitive wellbeing.

6. **Celebrating Your Progress:** We urge you to celebrate your accomplishments along the way, no matter how big or small. It's an amazing accomplishment to improve your brain health, and this cookbook is here to help you every step of the way.

So, keep in mind that you're doing more than just cooking when you open the pages of "Mind Diet Cookbook 2024" and peruse the culinary treats; you're also nourishing your brain, promoting mental clarity, and taking an essential step toward a more promising, vibrant future. Here is where your path to better brain health begins, and we are honored to walk it with you.

Chapter 1: The Foundations of the Mind Diet

In this introductory chapter, we set out on a quest to learn the fundamental ideas behind the Mind Diet, which serves as the cornerstone of our culinary research. The secret to realizing the full benefits of this dietary strategy for cognitive wellbeing is to comprehend these ideas. Here is a sample of what you will learn:

The Science Behind the Mind Diet

In this section, we delve into the intriguing research that supports the Mind Diet and present persuasive evidence for its ability to enhance cognitive health, lower the risk of cognitive decline, and prevent neurodegenerative disorders. The Mind Diet's scientific foundation is examined in more detail below:

1. **Nutrient-Rich Foods and Cognitive Health:** Examine the connection between nutrient-dense diets and mental health. Learn how diets rich in vitamins, minerals, antioxidants, and other key elements can crucially promote brain function.

2. **The Role of Antioxidants:** Examine the role that antioxidants have in the Mind Diet. Learn how these potent substances counteract inflammation and oxidative stress, two important elements linked to cognitive decline. Discover which foods are high in antioxidants and why they're so important for preserving brain health.

3. **Omega-3 Fatty Acids and Brain Function:** Find out how omega-3 fatty acids, in particular DHA and EPA, affect brain function significantly. Examine the research that suggests these fatty acids are essential for maintaining cognitive function and preventing cognitive problems.

4. **Inflammation and Cognitive Decline:** Learn more about the relationship between inflammatory aging and cognitive decline. Learn how the Mind Diet's focus on foods that fight inflammation can help lower the risk of neurodegenerative conditions like Alzheimer's and Parkinson's.

5. **Neuroplasticity and Mind Diet:** Learn about the idea of neuroplasticity or the brain's capacity for self-rewiring and adaptation. Investigate how the Mind Diet promotes neuroplasticity, possibly improving memory, learning, and cognitive flexibility.

6. **Real-World Evidence:** Enjoy real-world success stories and scientific studies that demonstrate the Mind Diet's beneficial effects on cognitive wellbeing. These experiences and studies offer solid proof of how this eating strategy might result in observable enhancements in brain function.

Key Nutrients for a Healthy Brain

We'll look at the vital nutrients in this part that serve as the foundation for a healthy, resilient brain. The Mind Diet's capacity to improve cognitive performance and advance general brain health is built on a foundation of these essential nutrients. The main nutrients you'll find are as follows:

1. **Omega-3 Fatty Acids**: Learn everything there is to know about omega-3 fatty acids, especially DHA and EPA (eicosatetraenoic acid). Learn how these vital lipids, which are frequently present in fatty fish like salmon, sardines, and trout, are crucial for preserving the structure and function of brain cells. Learn how to include foods high in omega-3s in your diet to enhance your memory and mental flexibility.

2. **Antioxidants:** Learn about the foods that are high in antioxidants that can shield your brain from inflammation and oxidative stress. Vitamin C, vitamin E, and other phytochemical antioxidants, which are present in colored fruits and vegetables, protect brain cells. Learn how to employ these antioxidant powerhouses in delectable recipes.

3. **Vitamin B:** Learn more about the B-vitamin family, which also includes B6, B9 (folate), and B12. By controlling homocysteine levels and assisting in the creation of neurotransmitters, these vitamins are essential for maintaining brain health. Find out where to get B vitamins in your diet and how they affect your mental health.

4. **Vitamin D:** Recognize the role of vitamin D in maintaining brain health and how it affects mood regulation and neuroprotection. Discover the greatest dietary sources of vitamin D and how to make sure you're getting the recommended amount each day.

5. **Minerals:** Examine the function of minerals like iron, zinc, and magnesium in the brain. Learn how these minerals contribute to the creation of memories, the

production of neurotransmitters, and general cognitive function.

6. **Polyphenols and Phytochemicals:** Enjoy the world of phytochemicals and polyphenols, which may be found in foods like green tea, dark chocolate, and berries. These substances are beneficial friends in maintaining cognitive function because of their strong anti-inflammatory and antioxidant capabilities.

Incorporating Mind Diet Principles into Your Daily Life

This part fills the gap between theory and practice by providing you with practical tips for incorporating Mind Diet ideas into your regular activities. You'll find helpful advice to incorporate a brain-boosting diet into your daily life, whether you're an experienced practitioner or brand-new to the idea:

- **Meal Planning Made Simple:** Learn how to easily plan your meals to adhere to the Mind Diet's principles. We'll help you develop balanced, brain-healthy diets that suit your dietary requirements and preferences. Difficulties with meals are over; welcome to stress-free, brain-nourishing dining.

- **Shopping for Brain-Healthy Ingredients:** As we offer advice for choosing the freshest and most nutrient-dense ingredients, you may shop with confidence. Learn how to recognize Mind Diet requirements and include them on your grocery list so you always have the ingredients for meals that will improve your brain function available.

- **The Art of Mindful Eating:** Discover the benefits of mindful eating and how it can change the way you feel about food. Learn how mindfulness can help healthy portion control, better digestion, and increase the enjoyment of meals. We'll provide useful tips for developing mindful eating practices.

- **Culinary Creativity with Mind Diet:** With recipes influenced by the Mind Diet, unleash your inner chef and use your imagination. In addition to exciting your taste sensations, we'll offer cooking advice and methods that enhance the nutritional value of products. You'll find culinary ideas for every occasion, from breakfast to dessert.

- **Social and Dining Out:** Follow the Mind Diet guidelines while navigating social gatherings and eating out. Learn how to convey your dietary preferences clearly and how to make brain-healthy decisions when you aren't in charge of the menu. Enjoy your social life while pursuing your objectives for cognitive wellbeing.

- **Building a Supportive Environment:** Establish a setting that supports your dedication to the Mind Diet. We'll talk about ways to organize your kitchen, storage ideas, and equipment that make preparing meals easier and promote healthier eating habits. Culinary delights that stimulate the brain might find a home in your kitchen.

Chapter 2: Breakfasts for Brainpower

Greetings on this lovely voyage through the realm of breakfasts that improve brain function. In this chapter, we'll look at a variety of breakfast foods that not only excite your taste buds but also give your brain the vital nutrients it needs to start the day with vigor and clarity. Here is a preview of what this chapter will cover:

Energizing Morning Smoothies

This section delves into the world of energizing morning smoothies—nutrient-rich elixirs created to give you a boost of energy and mental clarity as you start your day. These smoothies are not only delicious but also full of elements that stimulate the brain. You might discover some energizing recipes below:

Berry Blast Smoothie

- bright berries packed in antioxidants.
- Greek yogurt for protein and creaminess
- Kale or spinach for additional vitamins and minerals.
- A little honey for organic sweetness

Green Goddess Smoothie

- a lush combination of kale or spinach-like leafy greens
- Avocado cream for good fats
- pineapple with bananas for sweetness naturally
- For hydration, add a splash of coconut water.

Nutty Almond Delight

- A serving of creamy almond butter with healthful fats
- Bananas are naturally sweet and high in potassium.
- spinach to add additional nutrients.
- Almond milk provides a nutty flavor.

Tropical Sunrise Smoothie

- a mango, pineapple, and kiwi tropical fusion
- Greek yogurt provides probiotics and creaminess.
- Kale or spinach for an increase in nutrition
- Ginger for a zingy kick and a hint of it

Peanut Butter Power Smoothie

- Rich and flavorful peanut butter with added protein
- Bananas provide potassium and natural sweetness.
- Kale or spinach for additional nutrition.
- Greek yogurt provides probiotics and creaminess.

Every smoothie is thoughtfully made to offer a revitalizing, nutrient-rich start to your day. These morning elixirs are not only delectable but also aid in your efforts to achieve cognitive wellness because they are brimming with vitamins, minerals, antioxidants, and healthy fats. These invigorating morning smoothies have you covered whether you're looking for a creamy, nutty treat or an antioxidant boost from berry-infused foods. Prepare to sip your way to an improved morning and a more alert mind!

Wholesome Oatmeal Variations

In this section, we explore the comforting world of oatmeal, showcasing a diverse range of recipes that transform this humble grain into satisfying breakfasts brimming with brain-boosting nutrients. Whether you prefer the classic oatmeal or crave adventurous flavors, these variations offer something for every palate. Here's a taste of what you'll find:

Classic Comfort Oatmeal

- Rolling oats are a traditional favorite.
- warm seasonings like nutmeg and cinnamon
- toppings like raw almonds, fresh berries, and honey drizzle
- A cozy and wholesome start to your day

Apple Cinnamon Oatmeal

- Cinnamon is sautéed with fresh apples to provide a flavorful topping.
- For a hearty texture, use steel-cut oats.
- Add a few chopped walnuts or pecans for some crunching.
- A warm, comfortable breakfast that is inspired by fall.

Tropical Paradise Oatmeal

- Coconut milk that is creamy for a tropical twist
- pieces of pineapple for a dash of freshness
- For a Hawaiian flair, add coconut and macadamia nuts to the dish.
- A memorable oatmeal encounter.

Chocolate-Banana Oatmeal

- Mashable bananas and rich cocoa powder provide sweetness.
- Oats that have been rolled for a cozy feel.
- A generous sprinkle of almond butter
- A guilt-free breakfast that tastes like dessert.

Savory Spinach and Mushroom Oatmeal

- Adding a savory flavor with sautéed spinach and mushrooms
- The broth is made from vegetables or chicken for a richer flavor.
- Parmesan cheese sprinkled on top for umami goodness.
- Oatmeal with a spicy, brain-boosting twist

These oatmeal varieties are not only mouthwatering, but they are also loaded with vital vitamins, minerals, and fiber that support brain health. Every version of comfort oatmeal, whether you prefer the warmth of traditional comfort oatmeal or the exotic attraction of coconut and pineapple, offers a healthy and caring way to start your day with mental clarity and enduring vitality.

Brain-Boosting Breakfast Bowls

This section delves into the realm of brain-boosting breakfast bowls, colorful, wholesome concoctions that give you a filling, enticing start to the day. These bowls are made to whet your appetite and supply vital nutrients to help with cognitive function. You can discover the following delicious breakfast bowl variations:

Acai Berry Bliss Bowl

- Pureed acai berries for their antioxidant content and vibrant color.
- toppings like chia seeds, granola, and banana slices
- A tropical twist with coconut flakes and a drizzle of honey
- A revitalizing and energizing morning treat

Quinoa and Fruit Medley Bowl

- the use of quinoa, a source of protein
- A luscious explosion with sliced kiwi and other berries
- Greek yogurt for richness and probiotics, a spoonful
- Add some chopped nuts for extra crunch and good fats.

Chia Pudding Power Bowl

- Almond milk is used to make a creamy chia pudding.
- Sliced almonds, fresh berries, and a faint vanilla extract
- Pour some maple syrup on top for some natural sweetness.
- A filling and wholesome breakfast bowl

Greek Yogurt Parfait Bowl

- Greek yogurt thick as the foundation
- Berries, granola, and honey layers
- Add some hemp or flax seeds for more omega-3s.
- A delicious treat with lots of protein.

Sweet Potato and Nut Butter Bowl

- Cubes of roasted sweet potato for a different spin
- Nut butter for richness, such as almond or peanut
- Banana slices with a dash of cinnamon

- A warming and filling bowl of breakfast food

Every breakfast bowl is a work of art, fusing flavors, colors, and textures to stimulate the senses and fill the mind. Choose from the vivacious Acai Berry Bliss Bowl or the filling Quinoa and Fruit Medley Bowl; both are brimming with nutrients that enhance cognitive wellness while tantalizing your taste buds. Prepare to enjoy the pleasure of a visually attractive and nutrient-dense breakfast dish as you begin your day.

Nutrient-Packed Pancake Delights

With a healthy twist, we're honoring the cozy and pleasant world of pancakes in this section. These nutrient-dense pancake recipes are not only mouthwatering, but they also offer important nutrients to assist your mental health. These pancakes will make your day happier whether you eat them as a treat during the week or on a lazy weekend morning. Here is a sample of what you will discover:

Whole Grain Banana Pancakes

- mashed banana and whole wheat flour for added fiber and sweetness.
- A little vanilla essence and cinnamon for flavor
- Greek yogurt or pure maple syrup drizzled on top.
- A filling and healthy pancake option

Blueberry and Flaxseed Pancakes

- For antioxidants and a splash of freshness, use fresh blueberries.
- Omega-3 fatty acids are added by grinding flaxseed.

15

- Yogurt with a dollop and a touch of honey for richness
- A tasty fusion of flavor and nutrients that are good for the brain.

Spinach and Feta Savory Pancakes

- For a savory variation, add sautéed spinach and crumbled feta cheese.
- herb-infused whole grain pancake batter.
- Greek yogurt or a sprinkling of Parmesan cheese as a garnish
- An option for savory pancakes with a Mediterranean flavor

Pumpkin Spice Pancakes

- pumpkin puree from a can with toasty spices for a flavor of fall
- for more fiber, use whole wheat flour.
- Greek yogurt with a dollop and chopped pecans on top
- A warm and wholesome pancake option

Cocoa and Almond Butter Pancakes

- Almond butter and cocoa powder for a rich, chocolaty flavor
- Banana hints for a touch of natural sweetness
- For the garnish, add some honey and sliced almonds.
- a way to indulge in the delights of chocolate and nuts without feeling bad.

The critical vitamins, minerals, and good fats in these nutrient-dense pancakes provide your brain with a delicious way to start the day. Each recipe is a celebration of flavor and mental health, whether you opt for the comfort of Whole Grain Banana Pancakes or the decadence of Cocoa and Almond Butter Pancakes. Prepare to flip your way to a more contented, healthy mind!

Chapter 3: Lunches to Fuel Your Focus

We're glad you're here because this chapter will help you prepare meals that will not only satisfy your hunger but also give you continuous energy and mental clarity for the remainder of the day. These lunchtime brain-boosters are created to help you stay alert, motivated, and focused. Here's a preview of what's to come:

Colorful Salad Creations

We delve into the realm of colorful, nutrient-dense salads in this section—lunchtime concoctions that are as appetizing to the eye as they are to the palate. These vibrant salads are created to boost your energy and attention while providing your brain with the necessary nutrients. The following recipes for delicious salads can liven up your lunch:

Mediterranean Quinoa Salad

- Quinoa as the basis is packed with nutrients.
- Cherry tomatoes, cucumbers, and bell peppers mixed.
- feta cheese with kalamata olives for taste
- The dish's finishing touch is a lemon-herb vinaigrette.

Asian-Inspired Rainbow Salad

- Red cabbage that is bright and crunchy
- Bell peppers, carrots, and snap peas in shredded form
- Almond slices with sesame seeds for crunch
- Adding umami with a ginger-soy dressing

Berry and Spinach Power Salad

- vibrant spinach leaves and a variety of berries
- Add toasted walnuts or pecans for more texture.
- Crumbled feta or goat cheese for richness
- For a sweet and tangy note, use a balsamic vinaigrette.

Southwest Fiesta Salad

- Corn, black beans, and avocado dice
- For color, use cherry tomatoes and red onions.
- Tofu or grilled chicken as a protein source
- For a zesty finish, add cilantro lime dressing.

Roasted Beet and Goat Cheese Salad

- Roasted beets for an earthy flavor and bright color
- Arugula and mixed greens for a spicy bite
- Richness is provided by candied pecans and creamy goat cheese.
- A honey-Dijon sauce for a pleasing balance.

These vibrant salad creations give a nutrient-rich, tasty lunch experience in addition to being a visual feast. These salads are made to keep you energized and focused throughout the day, whether you select the Southwest Fiesta Salad with its robust and spicy undertones or the Mediterranean Quinoa Salad with its Mediterranean flair. Prepare to embrace the art of satisfying lunch salads that improve your cognitive fitness.

Hearty Grain-Based Lunches

This section examines filling, nutrient-dense grain-based lunches that keep your focus sharp all day long and provide you lasting energy. These dishes use a range of healthy grains as the base and combine them with a variety of colorful veggies, lean proteins, and savory herbs and spices. Here is a sample of what you will discover:

Quinoa and Chickpea Power Bowl

- the use of quinoa, a source of protein
- Chickpeas for more fiber and protein
- roasted vegetables such as broccoli and sweet potatoes
- A creamy and nutty dressing made with tahini.

Brown Rice and Teriyaki Tofu Stir-Fry

- As the foundation of the stir-fry, nutty brown rice
- Teriyaki sauce-marinated pieces of crispy tofu.
- a vibrant stir-fry with carrots, snow peas, and bell peppers
- To add some umami and savory flavor, use sesame ginger sauce.

Farro and Mediterranean Veggie Delight

- Featuring chewy, nutty farro as the main ingredient
- Mediterranean-inspired grilled bell peppers, zucchini, and eggplant
- Olives, feta cheese, and cherry tomatoes add flavor.
- An herb dressing with lemon for a bright, tangy finish

Spicy Lentil and Brown Rice Pilaf

- Brown rice and brown lentils for a hearty pilaf

- A blend of aromatic spices like cumin and paprika
- Sautéed onions, garlic, and bell peppers for depth of flavor
- A drizzle of yogurt or tzatziki for cooling contrast

Barley and Roasted Vegetable Bowl

- barley as the base is nutrient-dense.
- a variety of roasted veggies, including butternut squash and Brussels sprouts
- For a gourmet touch, use rich feta cheese or creamy goat cheese.
- For a sweet and tangy note, use a balsamic reduction.

These filling grain-based meals are made to keep you full, content, and energized for a successful day. Whether you choose the Farro and Mediterranean Veggie Delight with its Mediterranean flair or the Quinoa and Chickpea Power Bowl with its plant-based protein, each meal is a filling and nourishing choice that supports cognitive wellness while titillating your taste senses. Prepare to savor lunches that will not only satisfy your hunger but also sharpen your focus.

Vibrant Veggie Wraps and Sandwiches

The world of colorful vegetarian wraps and sandwiches—delicious and transportable lunch options that are stuffed with fresh veggies and components that are good for the brain—is something we delve into in this section. These dishes are ideal for anyone who needs a tasty and healthy lunch on the run. Here is a sample of what you will discover:

Hummus and Veggie Wrap

- Hummus as the foundation spread, creamy.
- A mixture of vibrant carrots, cucumbers, and bell peppers
- For more greens, use fresh spinach or arugula.
- Using a whole-grain tortilla, create a filling wrap.

Avocado and Chickpea Salad Sandwich

- Chickpeas and avocado are mashed together for smoothness and protein.
- Sliced red onion and tomato for freshness.
- For extra crunch, leafy greens like lettuce or baby spinach.
- Using whole-grain bread to make a healthy sandwich.

Grilled Vegetable Panini

- grilled vegetables including red onion, zucchini, and eggplant.
- For richness, use sliced mozzarella or a vegan cheese substitute.
- Fresh basil leaves for a flavorful explosion
- A warm and filling sandwich on a pressed whole-grain panini.

Greek Tzatziki Wrap

- Homemade tzatziki sauce with cucumber and Greek yogurt
- Red onion, cherry tomatoes, and cucumber slices
- For protein, broil some sliced tofu or chicken.
- A whole-wheat wrap makes a light and satisfying supper.

Portobello Mushroom and Pesto Sandwich

- Pesto-marinated Portobello mushroom caps, grilled or roasted.
- roasted red bell peppers in slices and young spinach.
- Balsamic glaze is drizzled on top for a sweet and tangy finish.
- A ciabatta roll makes a filling and upscale sandwich.

In addition to being visually pleasing, these colorful vegetarian wraps and sandwiches offer a delicious variety of tastes and sensations. Whether you opt for the Grilled Vegetable Panini with its smokey grilled vegetables or the Hummus and Veggie Wrap with its creamy hummus goodness, these dishes are made to offer a filling and time-saving lunch that will keep you motivated all day. Prepare to embrace the art of enhancing your cognitive wellness with a veggie-centric meal.

Soups and Stews for Mental Clarity

We go into the realm of hearty, savory soups, and stews in this part, which will not only warm your spirit but also give you the critical nutrients you need to improve your concentration and attention. These dishes would make a filling and stimulating meal. Here is a sample of what you will discover:

Butternut Squash and Sage Soup

- a silky base made from pureed, creamy butternut squash.
- Sage leaves with a delicate scent for an earthy note.
- A sprinkling of roasted pumpkin seeds and a drizzle of olive oil

- A warming soup that calms the senses and stimulates the intellect.

Chicken and Vegetable Quinoa Stew

- Tender chicken breasts or a plant-based protein substitute
- a variety of vibrant veggies, including bell peppers, carrots, and celery
- Quinoa is nutrient-dense for extra heartiness.
- A cozy stew in a flavorful broth with herbs and spices

Tomato and Basil Bisque

- Fresh basil and ripe tomatoes for a flavorful explosion
- Greek yogurt or creamy coconut milk for richness
- Balsamic reduction is tossed in for a sweet and tangy finish.
- A traditional soup with a modern touch to promote mental clarity.

Lentil and Spinach Curry Soup

- Red lentils for fiber and plant-based protein
- For a nutritional boost, use diced tomatoes and spinach leaves.
- a flavorful curry mixture with savory spices
- a filling soup with flavor that helps you concentrate.

Mushroom and Barley Broth

- Sautéed mushrooms for an earthy and umami depth
- Chewy and nutty barley for added texture and fiber.
- A blend of herbs and a splash of white wine
- A comforting and nourishing broth that enhances mental clarity.

These stews and soups are not only delectable and warming, but they also offer a wealth of minerals and elements that are good for the brain. These dishes are made to keep you focused, energized, and cognitively sharp throughout the day, whether you select the butternut squash and sage soup with its silky texture or the tomato and basil bisque with its vivid tastes. Prepare to enjoy the deliciousness of stews and soups that improve your mental health.

Chapter 4: Dinner Delights for Cognitive Vitality

We examine a selection of evening treats in this chapter that are not only delicious but also designed to maintain and improve cognitive health. These dishes are created to please your taste senses after a hard day by providing your brain with important nutrients and spices. Here is a sample of the culinary gems you will find:

Poultry and Seafood Specials

We dig into a world of delectable seafood and poultry recipes in this section. The essential nutrients from lean proteins and omega-3 fatty acids in these meals are chosen to deliver a delicious supper experience while supporting cognitive wellbeing. Here is a sample of what you will learn:

Lemon-Herb Roasted Chicken

- savory chicken that has been seasoned with a variety of fresh herbs.
- Lemon zesty for flavor and brightness.
- served with quinoa pilaf and roasted veggies.
- a traditional chicken dish that has been improved for mental health.

Garlic Butter Shrimp Scampi

- Sautéed in butter with garlic, plump shrimp.
- Combined with zucchini or angel hair pasta.

- sprinkled with Parmesan cheese and fresh parsley as a garnish.
- A seafood treat that satisfies cravings and promotes brain health.

Baked Salmon with Dill and Asparagus

- Salmon fillets with a dill and lemon marinade cooked in the oven.
- Perfectly grilled spears of tender asparagus.
- served as a complete dinner with couscous or quinoa.
- A delicious fish dish rich in omega-3s

Turkey and Spinach Stuffed Bell Peppers

- spinach, ground turkey, and flavorful seasonings.
- stuffed with filling, then baked in vibrant bell peppers.
- served with a side of broccoli or a salad.
- a nourishing, protein-rich dinner that promotes mental health.

Grilled Swordfish with Mango Salsa

- Perfectly cooked swordfish steaks that have been marinated.
- Add a colorful mango salsa on top.
- Served with a dish of quinoa or wild rice.
- a mouthwatering seafood experience that stimulates the brain.

Each recipe in this section aims to provide a wonderful dining experience while maximizing the benefits of seafood and lean poultry for your cognitive fitness. These recipes are certain to satisfy your palette and energize your mind, whether you select the Lemon-Herb Roasted Chicken for its zesty and herbaceous flavors or the Garlic Butter Shrimp Scampi for its decadent seafood charm. Prepare to enjoy the greatest seafood and poultry specialties for dinner.

Plant-Based Power Dinners

With a selection of filling and healthy dinners, we highlight the flavors and health advantages of plant-based eating in this section. The richness of plant-based nutrients in these meals encourages cognitive wellness while creating a delicious supper experience. Here is a sample of what you will discover:

Chickpea and Vegetable Curry

- wholesome chickpeas and a variety of vibrant vegetables
- in a flavorful and aromatic curry sauce simmered.
- served with fresh naan bread or over brown rice.
- a supper powered by plants that nourish the body and the soul.

Portobello Mushroom Steaks

- Perfectly marinated and grilled meaty Portobello mushroom caps.
- with a flavorful herb and garlic sauce on top.
- served with a dish of roasted sweet potatoes or quinoa.
- A filling and umami-rich dinner to support mental health.

Lentil and Sweet Potato Stew

- Sweet potatoes with nutrient-dense lentils in a filling stew
- seasoned with paprika and cumin, two warming spices.
- Fresh lemon juice squeezed for brightness.

- a warming stew made of plants that promote mental clarity.

Vegan Eggplant Parmesan

- Sweet potatoes with nutrient-dense lentils in a filling stew
- seasoned with paprika and cumin, two warming spices.
- Fresh lemon juice squeezed for brightness.
- a warming stew made of plants that promote mental clarity.

Quinoa-Stuffed Bell Peppers

- Nutty quinoa mixed with a variety of herbs and veggies.
- stuffed with filling, then baked in vibrant bell peppers.
- balsamic reduction drizzled on top for a hint of sweetness.
- A wholesome and protein-rich plant-based dinner that fuels your focus.

Each plant-based power dinner in this section is designed to offer a satisfying and nourishing dining experience while harnessing the benefits of plant-based ingredients for cognitive wellness. Whether you choose the Chickpea and Vegetable Curry for its rich flavors or the Vegan Eggplant Parmesan for its Italian-inspired goodness, these recipes are sure to please your palate and support your cognitive vitality. Get ready to enjoy the best of plant-based power for dinner.

Satisfying Grains and Legumes

In this part, we examine a mouthwatering selection of recipes that emphasize the healthful goodness of grains and legumes. These dishes are designed to nurture your cognitive wellness while giving you a hearty and delicious supper experience. They do this by utilizing the benefits of complex carbs and plant-based proteins. Here is an example of some of the healthy creations you can find:

Lentil and Brown Rice Pilaf

- Brown rice and lentils for a basis that is high in fiber.
- fragrant spice mixture for taste depth
- onions, garlic, and vibrant bell peppers sautéed.
- A nutritious and flavorful pilaf that promotes mental health.

Quinoa and Black Bean Enchiladas

- Black beans and protein-rich quinoa serve as the stuffing.
- filled with enchilada sauce and rolled into corn tortillas.
- optionally topped with dairy cheese or vegan cheese.
- A tasty and filling meal with Mexican influences.

Barley and Mushroom Risotto

- Barley grains that are perfectly chewy and creamy cooked
- Mushrooms and shallots sautéed for a rich umami flavor.
- A little white wine and some chopped fresh herbs
- A warm and filling risotto that will thrill your brain.

Chickpea and Vegetable Stir-Fry

- Yummy, tender chickpeas and a rainbow of vibrant vegetables
- Using ginger soy sauce and flavorful garlic in a stir-fry
- served as a complete meal with brown rice or quinoa.
- A flavorful stir-fry made of plants that satisfy the appetite and the mind.

Wild Rice and Cranberry Stuffed Acorn Squash

- Tart cranberries paired with nutty wild rice.
- into roasted acorn squash halves stuffed.
- Finished with a delicious coating of maple balsamic.
- A delicious dish with remarkable visual appeal that promotes cognitive wellness.

These substantial dinners made of grains and legumes are intended to offer a gratifying and nutrient-rich dining experience. These recipes are certain to satisfy your palette while fueling your intellect, whether you choose the Quinoa and Black Bean Enchiladas for their Mexican flair or the Wild Rice and Cranberry Stuffed Acorn Squash for their elegance. Prepare to savor cozy and nourishing meals that will enhance your mental health.

Flavorful Mindful Desserts

This section explores the world of sweets, which are not only delectable but also mindfully created to promote your cognitive fitness. These dessert recipes are created to sate your sweet needs while integrating tastes and nutrients that are good for the brain. Here's a sample of the delicious treats you may expect to find:

Dark Chocolate Avocado Mousse

- Richness is added by blending creamy avocado with dark chocolate.
- a little bit of honey or maple syrup added for sweetness.
- Fresh berries and chopped almonds are used as decorations.

- A delicious dessert full of antioxidants for the pleasure of the brain

Berry-Infused Chia Pudding

- Chia seeds steeped in almond milk with berry flavoring.
- Finished with a honey drizzle and a variety of fresh berries on top.
- For texture, add some toasted coconut flakes.
- A pudding that is both healthy and guilt-free for sweet delight

Baked Apple Crisp with Oat Topping

- Apples are cut into slices and spiced with cinnamon and nutmeg.
- topped with a filling crumble of oats and almonds.
- heated and accompanied by a dollop of Greek yogurt or a dairy-free substitute.
- a nourishing dessert that's high in fiber and helps mental health.

Nut Butter Banana Ice Cream

- For smoothness, frozen bananas were mixed with nut butter.
- Vanilla extract was used for flavor.
- Finished with sliced bananas and honey or date syrup drizzle.
- Dairy-free and decadent, this delicacy will thrill your brain.

Lemon-Berry Yogurt Parfait

- Greek yogurt or dairy-free yogurt layers that are tart.

- For brightness and sweetness, add some fresh lemon zest and berry compote.
- For crunch, add some crushed nuts or granola.
- A tart and nutrient-dense parfait to sate your sweet tooth.

Each delectable dessert in this section celebrates both taste and mental health. These desserts are made to satisfy your sweet tooth while nourishing your brain, whether you choose the Dark Chocolate Avocado Mousse for its decadent chocolate richness or the Baked Apple Crisp with Oat Topping for its cozy warmth. Prepare yourself to savor desserts that are as delicious as they are attentive.

Chapter 5: Snacks and Sides that Nourish.

This chapter explores a wide range of delectable snacks and sides that not only tempt the palate but also supply vital nutrients to support cognitive fitness. These dishes are made to improve your general health and mental clarity, whether you're searching for a delectable lunchtime pick-me-up or a tasty side dish to your meals. Here's a taste of what delicious options you may expect to find:

Guilt-Free Snacking Options

We provide several guilt-free snacking options in this section so you can indulge your appetites without jeopardizing your mental health. These snacks are made to be both tasty and nourishing, giving you a filling snack that promotes mental clarity. Here are some examples of the healthy and guilt-free snack options you can find:

Crunchy Kale Chips

- Olive oil and sea salt are combined with fresh kale leaves.
- baked until perfectly crisp for a delicious crunch.
- a guilt-free method to eat greens in the shape of chips.

Greek Yogurt and Berries Parfait

- Fresh berries are placed on top of creamy Greek yogurt.
- sprinkle of maple syrup or honey for natural sweetness
- a protein- and anti-oxidant-rich parfait.

Spiced Almonds and Walnuts

- Walnuts and almonds toasted with a mixture of comforting spices.
- A tiny bit of honey to provide a touch of sweetness.
- A tasty and high-protein nut mixture for on-the-go munching.

Sliced Cucumber and Hummus

- Pairing creamy hummus with crunchy cucumber slices.
- A snack that is both hydrating and reviving
- a high-fiber, low-calorie option that is vitamin and fiber-rich.

Fresh Fruit Salad with a Citrus Zest

- seasonal fruit medley including melons, berries, and citrus.
- Citrus fruit juice and zest add a fresh and tangy edge.
- Fruit salad is rich in vitamins and flavor.

In addition to being delicious, these guilt-free snack choices offer vital nutrients to support your cognitive fitness. These snacks are made to fulfill appetites while feeding the brain, whether you choose the Spiced Almonds and Walnuts for their savory-spicy taste or the Crunchy Kale Chips for their pleasing crunch. Prepare to indulge in delightful, guilt-free munching that promotes mental clarity.

Fresh and Flavorful Sides

This section explores a delectable selection of savory side dishes that go well with your entrees and improve the dining experience. These sides are made with colorful ingredients to support your cognitive wellness while delivering a rush of flavor and nutrition. Here's an example of the tasty and reviving sides you'll encounter:

Caprese Salad with Balsamic Glaze

- Fresh mozzarella, ripe tomatoes, and basil leaves
- Served with a tart and sweet balsamic reduction on top.
- a traditional Italian side dish that is vibrant and flavorful.

Quinoa and Herb-Stuffed Bell Peppers

- Spices and herbs are used to prepare quinoa.
- stuffed with filling, then baked in vibrant bell peppers.
- A colorful, protein-rich side dish that is filling and healthy.

Roasted Asparagus with Lemon and Parmesan

- Perfectly grilled spears of tender asparagus.
- fresh lemon juice and zest for brightness
- Add some grated Parmesan cheese for a salty finishing touch.
- a tasty side dish that is very stylish.

Greek Tzatziki Cucumber Salad

- with red onion, cherry tomatoes, and sliced cucumbers
- Greek yogurt that is creamy and tart is added. Tzatziki dressing
- a light side dish with Mediterranean influences to go with your meals.

Mango and Black Bean Salsa

- Black beans, multicolored bell peppers, and diced mango
- For a flavorful kick, use a tangy lime and cilantro dressing.
- a spicy and sweet side dish that gives your meal a touch of the tropics.

Each delectable side dish in this section has been carefully created to offer a light and healthy touch to your meals. Whether you select the Mango and Black Bean Salsa for its tropical flair or the Caprese Salad for its traditional Italian charm, these sides are made to improve your dining experience while promoting cognitive vigor. Prepare to indulge in sides that will not only tempt your taste senses but also feed your brain.

Brain-Boosting Dips and Spreads

This section delves into the realm of tasty dips and spreads that enhance the flavor and cognitive health of your meals, snacks, and appetizers. Every swallow of these spreads and dips is designed to give you vital nutrients and flavor. Here are a few examples of the delectable and nutritious options you can choose from:

Guacamole with a Twist

- A creamy avocado, tomatoes, onions, and cilantro are combined.
- Adding a tiny bit of cayenne or jalapeno for a spicy kick
- An innovative take on the traditional guacamole will spice up you're snacking.

Nut Butter and Banana Spread

- ripe banana combined with nut butter, such as almond, peanut, or cashew.
- For natural sweetness, a little bit of honey or maple syrup
- a spread that goes well with fruit, porridge, or bread.

Roasted Red Pepper Hummus

- Garlic and roasted red peppers are combined with chickpeas.
- Olive oil drizzled and smoked paprika sprinkled.
- a flavorful, protein-rich hummus that is smokey and delicious.

Spinach and Artichoke Dip with a Healthy Twist

- Greek yogurt and cream cheese are used to make this delicious dip.
- Artichoke hearts, spinach, and a hint of nutmeg
- A more nutritious variation of the traditional dip that is great for sharing.

Walnut Pesto

- A colorful pesto made with walnuts and basil.
- For a cheesy touch, use nutritional yeast or parmesan cheese.
- Perfect as a savory dip, on pasta, or in sandwiches.

These cognitively enhancing dips and spreads not only improve your snacking and eating experiences but also give you the nutrients you need to maintain your mental health. Whether you select the Nut Butter & Banana Spread for its sweet and nutty richness or the Guacamole with a Twist for its spicy zing, these choices are made to satiate your palate while fueling your intellect. Prepare to savor spreads and dips that are tantalizing and beneficial to your mental clarity.

Homemade Nut Mixes and Trail Mixes

The world of handmade nut mixes and trail mixes, where creativity and nutrition come together to offer you scrumptious and invigorating snacks, is what we'll be exploring in this part. These mixes have been carefully created to offer a pleasing crunch and an increase in nutrients that benefit the brain. A sample of the delicious nut and trail mixtures you'll make is shown below:

Classic Nut Medley

- a combination of pecans, cashews, walnuts, and almonds
- Sea salt was added after a light roasting.
- A traditional favorite that's high in protein and good fats.

Tropical Paradise Trail Mix

- Flakes of coconut, mango, and dried pineapple.
- Banana chips, cashews, and macadamia nuts combined.
- The trail mix that takes you to the tropics is sweet and exotic.

Spicy Sriracha Almond Mix

- Roasted almonds seasoned with Sriracha.
- chickpeas or dried edamame for more crunch
- a nut with a blast of heat that is both spicy and flavorful.

Chocolate Lover's Trail Mix

- Dark chocolate chunks or almonds coated with chocolate.
- Combined with pretzels, dried cherries, and roasted almonds.

- a trail mix that satisfies your hunger for chocolate while being sweet and salty.

Mixed Mediterranean Olive and Nuts

- toasted almonds, pistachios, and green olives combined.
- seasoned with herbs and spices from the Mediterranean.
- A savory nut with a tinge of brininess that is inspired by the Mediterranean.

These handmade nut mixtures and trail mixes are great for mid-afternoon pick-me-ups, yogurt toppings, and on-the-go snacks. Whether you go for the Spicy Sriracha Almond Mix for its fiery kick or the Classic Nut Medley for its timelessness, these mixes are made to gratify your taste buds while maintaining your energy levels and mental clarity. Prepare to make delicious and beneficial nut and trail mixes that will help your cognitive fitness.

Chapter 6: Mind Diet for Special Occasions

In this chapter, we explore how the Mind Diet can be adapted to special occasions, allowing you to celebrate and indulge while still prioritizing cognitive wellness. These recipes are curated to provide a delightful and health-conscious approach to special events, gatherings, and celebrations. Here's a glimpse of the mouthwatering dishes and treats that will elevate your special occasions:

Hosting Brain-Healthy Parties

This section delves into the craft of throwing brain-healthy parties, where you may commemorate important events with delectable foods and sweets that put cognitive wellness first. These menu suggestions and dishes for parties have been carefully chosen to make your gathering both enjoyable and healthy for you and your guests. Here are some ideas for organizing events that are good for the brain:

Mindful Appetizer Spread

- Make an appetizer spread that is full of vibrant and healthy foods.
- Provide choices like hummus-topped fresh vegetable plates, whole-grain crackers with a selection of dipping sauces, and roasted nuts with herbs and spices.
- Invite your visitors to thoughtfully munch while mingling.

Brain-Boosting Beverages

- Serve alcoholic and anti-oxidant-rich beverages.
- Make herbal iced tea or sparkling water that has been infused with berries and herbs.
- Provide a variety of fresh fruit smoothies with components like blueberries and walnuts that have been shown to improve cognition.

Nourishing Main Course

- Select a main dish that features lean proteins and colorful vegetables.
- Think about dishes like quinoa salad with a variety of vegetables and a side of steaming greens, as well as herb-marinated grilled chicken or tofu skewers.
- To satisfy dietary restrictions, make sure you provide a vegetarian or vegan option.

Healthy Dessert Bar

- A dessert stand with brain-healthy foods should be set up.
- Include items like yogurt parfait stations with granola and almonds, strawberries coated in dark chocolate, and fruit skewers.
- Allow your guests to personalize their desserts to their liking.

Interactive Brain Games

- Play puzzles and games that are interactive and enjoyable at your party.
- Crossword puzzles, brainteasers, or memory-boosting games are good ways to test your guests.

- Cognitive exercises can improve mental acuity while also being interesting.

Mindfulness and Relaxation Corner

- Set up a quiet area for meditation and rest.
- Offer yoga mats, pillows for meditation, or sessions of supervised meditation.
- Encourage your visitors to relax and take a rest while the celebrations are going on.

You may arrange memorable and healthful events that promote cognitive wellness while honoring significant occasions with your loved ones by using these ideas and dishes for brain-healthy celebrations. These well-thought-out party ideas provide the ideal balance of mouthwatering flavors and options that will stimulate the mind, ensuring that everyone will have a fulfilling experience. Prepare to arrange celebrations that place a high priority on mental health.

Mind Diet for Holidays and Celebrations

In this section, we'll look at how to apply the Mind Diet's core principles to festive situations so that you can still put a high priority on your cognitive health. These Christmas menu suggestions and recipes have been carefully chosen to provide a mix of traditional and nutritious options. Here are some ideas for how to observe the holidays while keeping the Mind Diet in mind:

Festive Mindful Feast

- Create a Christmas spread that features a variety of dishes that will sharpen your mind.

- Serve a juicy roast turkey as the centerpiece or a vegetarian dish like stuffed acorn squash.
- Add colorful roasted veggies, quinoa salad, and a reduced-sugar cranberry chutney to the main dish to complete it.

Nutrient-Rich Holiday Sides

- By emphasizing healthy ingredients, you can elevate your holiday side dishes.
- A variety of greens sautéed with garlic and lemon, sweet potato mash with a hint of cinnamon, and whole-grain stuffing with nuts and dried fruits should be served.
- For enhanced flavor and beneficial effects on the brain, add herbs like rosemary and thyme.

Mindful Appetizers and Snacks

- Start your celebration with scrumptious nibbles and appetizers.
- A Mediterranean mezze plate, whole-grain crackers with olive tapenade, and a mixed nut assortment seasoned with herbs are just a few of the items you can provide.
- As your guests mingle, encourage them to munch on these snacks that are good for the brain.

Vibrant Holiday Desserts

- Desserts that are delicious and healthy are available.
- Prepare a fruit-focused dessert like a baked apple crisp with a nut topping or a berry trifle with Greek yogurt.
- Reduce additional sugars and rely more on fruit's natural sweetness and a little honey or maple syrup.

Mindful Eating Rituals

- When you are celebrating the holidays, promote mindfulness.
- Give thanks and take a minute to ponder before the meal.
- Encourage savoring each meal and spending time with loved ones while eating slowly and mindfully.

Active Holiday Traditions

- Make sure to get some exercise throughout the holidays.
- Plan a family trip or walk, participate in outdoor activities, or watch a friendly sporting event.
- Keeping active over the holidays encourages mental and physical wellness.

During holidays and celebrations, you can enjoy the tastes of the season while making decisions that promote your cognitive wellness by adhering to the Mind Diet principles. These holiday suggestions and menus strike a balance between joyous excess and conscientious healthfulness, guaranteeing that you can make priceless memories while caring for your brain. Prepare to celebrate the holidays with joy and with mental clarity.

Incorporating Mindful Eating into Social Gatherings

We explore mindful eating in this section, including how to apply it to social situations and events. By encouraging us to be mindful and fully immerse ourselves in the flavors and sensations of our meals, mindful eating increases both enjoyment and awareness. The following advice can help you incorporate mindful eating into your social interactions:

Setting the Stage:

- With sufficient seats and lighting, create a warm and cozy dining atmosphere.
- To improve the meal experience, arrange a beautifully set table with attention to detail, including tableware and centerpieces.

Mindful Moments:

- Start the gathering with a brief period of reflection or thanks.
- Encourage your guests to take a moment, relax, and thank you for the food and each other's company.

Engaging the Senses:

- Encourage your guests to enjoy their food with all their senses.
- Before they take their first mouthful, instruct them to take a moment to appreciate the foods' hues, textures, and scents.

Slow and Savory Bites:

- Encourage everyone to take their time and enjoy each meal.
- To properly savor many dishes and flavors, encourage smaller servings.

Mindful Conversation:

- Encourage thoughtful discussion about food and the dining experience.
- Encourage your visitors to express their sentiments and opinions about the tastes and sensations they are tasting.

Reducing Distractions:

- Distractions during the meal, such as loud background noise or electronic gadgets, should be kept to a minimum.
- Establish a setting that promotes deep and focused connections.

Appreciating Variety:

- Provide a wide range of foods to suit various palates and preferences.
- Encourage your guests to enjoy the variety of flavors and try new items.

Moderation and Balance:

- Emphasize the importance of moderation and balance in eating.
- Remind your guests that it's okay to enjoy indulgent treats in moderation while savoring healthier options as well.

Dessert Delights:

- Encourage people to eat dessert consciously, focusing only on the pleasure and satisfaction it provides.
- Encourage your guests to share dessert and enjoy it together.

Gratitude and Reflection:

- Finish the gathering with a moment of thanks and introspection.
- Request thanks from your guests for the meal, the companionship, and the thoughtful experience.

The way we view food and share meals in social settings can be changed by incorporating mindful eating. You may develop a stronger connection between food and the moments you enjoy with your visitors by encouraging them to be present, savor every meal, and converse with one another. This will enhance both your social and gastronomic experiences.

Chapter 7: Weekly Meal Plans and Grocery Lists

We go into the application of the Mind Diet in this chapter by giving you weekly meal plans and corresponding grocery lists. These menu plans provide you with a planned and practical method for meal preparation, which is intended to make your road toward cognitive wellness easier. An example of what to anticipate from this chapter is given below:

Meal Planning Made Easy

We've streamlined the meal planning procedure in this part to make it convenient and effective on your journey toward cognitive wellness. The Mind Diet principles can be followed while ensuring that your meals are satisfying and fulfilling with the help of meal planning. Here is a step-by-step tutorial for simple meal planning:

1. Set Your Goals:

- We've streamlined the meal planning procedure in this part to make it convenient and effective on your journey toward cognitive wellness. The Mind Diet principles can be followed while ensuring that your meals are satisfying and fulfilling with the help of meal planning. Here is a step-by-step tutorial for simple meal planning:

2. Choose Your Timeframe:

- Choose the time frame over which you wish to arrange your meals. Depending on your schedule and interests, you can choose a weekly, biweekly, or even monthly planning schedule.

3. Create a Master List:

- Make a list of your preferred Mind Diet components and dishes. This should be your go-to source for meal planning.

4. Select Your Recipes:

- Pick a collection of dishes that fit your dietary requirements and goals. A good selection of breakfast, lunch, supper, and snack alternatives is important.

5. Build Your Weekly Menu:

- Create a menu for the coming week using a blank weekly meal planner template or a computer program. Set aside particular recipes for each day.

6. Check Your Pantry:

- Check your cupboard, fridge, and freezer for ingredients you already have before generating a grocery list. This prevents making pointless purchases.

7. Create a Grocery List:

- Make a thorough grocery list based on the meals you plan to serve each day. To make your shopping easier, group the list by food types (such as fruits, vegetables, grains, and proteins).

8. Shop with Purpose:

- Stick to your list when shopping and refrain from making impulsive purchases. Concentrate on choosing high-quality, fresh foods.

9. Prep Ahead:

- Set aside a set day or hour to prepare meals. To make cooking over the week more convenient, prepare snacks in advance and chop veggies and proteins for marinating.

10. Be Flexible:

- Recognize that life is unpredictable. Be willing to modify your menu as necessary, whether because of unforeseen timetable changes or changes in ingredient supply.

11. Mindful Eating:

- Practice mindful eating by taking your time with each bite, appreciating the flavors and textures, and paying attention to your body's signals of hunger and fullness.

12. Track and Adjust:

- Keep track of your meals and any significant changes in your mood. Utilize this input to modify your future meal plans.

You can make meal planning easier by using these tips to make it a doable and pleasurable part of your daily routine. Meal planning not only makes it easier to follow the Mind Diet guidelines, but it also guarantees that you consistently feed your body and mind nourishing, delicious meals. Prepare to set out on a journey of thoughtful and nourishing eating thanks to the effectiveness of simple meal planning.

Shopping for Mind Diet Success

We delve into the art of Mind Diet success buying in this part. Your grocery store decisions are extremely important for promoting cognitive wellness, and with the correct mindset, you can turn every trip into a step in the direction of a more alert mind and a fitter body. Here are some crucial pointers for successful Mind Diet shopping:

Plan Your Shopping Trips:

- To ensure you have enough time to make thoughtful decisions, set aside particular times to go grocery shopping.
- Make a list of the ingredients and recipes you'll need in advance, keeping in mind the Mind Diet's guiding principles.

Embrace the Perimeter:

- Focus on purchasing items that are normally found along the store's perimeter, such as fresh produce, lean proteins, and whole grains.
- Spend as little time as possible in the central aisles, which frequently have processed and less healthy goods.

Prioritize Fresh Produce:

- Put a colorful assortment of fruits and veggies in your shopping cart. To provide a variety of nutrients, try to include a rainbow of hues.
- When possible, choose seasonal and locally farmed vegetables to provide the best freshness.

opt for Whole Grains:

- Instead of refined grains, choose whole grains such as whole wheat bread, brown rice, quinoa, and oats. Look for items with the phrase "100% whole grain" on the label.

Quality Protein Sources:

- Pick skinless poultry, fish, lentils, tofu, and lean meat cuts as your lean protein sources.
- For their omega-3 fatty acids, which are renowned for their advantages to the brain, think about including fatty fish like salmon and trout.

Include Nuts and Seeds:

- Add other nuts and seeds, like flaxseeds, chia seeds, almonds, and walnuts, to your shopping cart. These are full of important minerals and good fats.

Dairy or Dairy Alternatives:

- If you eat dairy, go for low- or no-fat varieties. To prevent additional sugars, choose unsweetened dairy substitutes.

Read Labels Mindfully:

- Read labels thoroughly before purchasing packaged foods. Look for items with few artificial additives, saturated fats, and added sugars.
- Pick products with fewer and recognized substances on the ingredient list.

Minimize Sugary and Processed Snacks:

- Limit your consumption of highly processed foods, sugary drinks, and snacks.

- Instead, pick healthy snacks like yogurt, fresh fruit, or homemade treats that adhere to the Mind Diet's tenets.

Stay Hydrated:

- Don't forget to drink water or herbal teas to stay hydrated. Limit your intake of sugary beverages and drink too much coffee.

Consider Frozen and Canned Options:

- Stock up on low-sodium canned products and frozen fruits and veggies. When fresh vegetables are hard to come by, these might be practical and healthy alternatives.

Bring Your Mindfulness:

- Focus on your list and your dietary objectives as you shop with mindfulness.
- To avoid making impulsive purchases of harmful snacks, avoid shopping when you are hungry.

You may turn your supermarket excursions into chances for Mind Diet success by implementing these shopping techniques. You'll not only feed your body and mind with thoughtful planning, but you'll also open the door to a brighter and more exciting future. Prepare to shop your way to gastronomic bliss and mental wellness.

Weekly Meal Plans for Your Brain Health

These weekly meal plans for supporting brain health are based on the ideas of the Mind Diet. These meal plans emphasize foods renowned for their cognitive advantages while offering a balanced mix of nutrients and flavors.

Weekly Meal Plan 1:

Day 1:

- Breakfast: Greek yogurt with berries and a sprinkle of almonds.
- Lunch: Spinach and quinoa salad with grilled chicken.
- Snack: Carrot sticks with hummus.
- Dinner: Baked salmon with steamed broccoli and quinoa.
- Dessert: Fresh fruit salad.

Day 2:

- Breakfast: Oatmeal with sliced banana and a drizzle of honey.
- Lunch: Whole-grain wrap with turkey, avocado, and mixed greens.
- Snack: Mixed nuts (almonds, walnuts, and cashews).
- Dinner: Stir-fried tofu with colorful bell peppers and brown rice.
- Dessert: Dark chocolate-covered strawberries.

Day 3:

- Breakfast: Scrambled eggs with sautéed spinach and tomatoes.
- Lunch: Lentil and vegetable soup with a side of whole-grain crackers.
- Snack: Sliced cucumber with tzatziki.
- Dinner: Grilled shrimp with quinoa and roasted asparagus.
- Dessert: Greek yogurt with honey and a sprinkle of cinnamon.

Day 4:

- Breakfast: Smoothie with kale, banana, blueberries, and flaxseeds.
- Lunch: Quinoa salad with chickpeas, cucumber, and feta cheese.
- Snack: Apple slices with almond butter.
- Dinner: Baked chicken breast with sweet potato and green beans.
- Dessert: Mixed berry parfait with Greek yogurt.

Day 5:

- Breakfast: Whole-grain toast with smashed avocado and a poached egg.
- Lunch: Mediterranean salad with mixed greens, olives, feta, and grilled chicken.
- Snack: Celery sticks with peanut butter.
- Dinner: Baked trout with a side of quinoa and steamed broccoli.
- Dessert: Sliced mango with a squeeze of lime.

Day 6:

- Breakfast: Cottage cheese with pineapple and a drizzle of honey.
- Lunch: Whole-grain pasta with tomato, basil, and grilled shrimp.
- Snack: Mixed berries.
- Dinner: Stir-fried lean beef with broccoli and brown rice.
- Dessert: Baked apple with cinnamon and a dollop of Greek yogurt.

Day 7:

- Breakfast: Whole-grain waffles with fresh strawberries and a dollop of yogurt.
- Lunch: Spinach and arugula salad with grilled salmon and a lemon vinaigrette.
- Snack: Trail mix with almonds, dried cranberries, and dark chocolate chips.
- Dinner: Roasted chicken with quinoa and roasted Brussels sprouts.
- Dessert: Sliced kiwi and a piece of dark chocolate.

Weekly Meal Plan 2:

Day 1:

- Breakfast: Overnight oats with sliced banana and chopped walnuts.
- Lunch: Spinach and berry salad with grilled chicken and a balsamic vinaigrette.
- Snack: Celery sticks with cream cheese.
- Dinner: Baked cod with quinoa and sautéed spinach.
- Dessert: Fresh pineapple chunks.

Day 2:

- Breakfast: Scrambled eggs with diced tomatoes and a sprinkle of feta cheese.
- Lunch: Lentil and vegetable stir-fry with tofu.
- Snack: Mixed nuts (almonds, cashews, and pistachios).
- Dinner: Grilled turkey burgers with a side of sweet potato fries and steamed broccoli.

- Dessert: Greek yogurt with a drizzle of honey and sliced strawberries.

Day 3:

- Breakfast: Smoothie with kale, banana, blueberries, and a spoonful of almond butter.
- Lunch: Quinoa salad with chickpeas, cucumber, and mint.
- Snack: Carrot sticks with hummus.
- Dinner: Baked salmon with quinoa and roasted asparagus.
- Dessert: Dark chocolate-covered blueberries.

Day 4:

- Breakfast: Whole-grain toast with smashed avocado and a poached egg.
- Lunch: Mediterranean wrap with grilled chicken, roasted red peppers, and tzatziki.
- Snack: Sliced apple with almond butter.
- Dinner: Stir-fried shrimp with brown rice and mixed vegetables.
- Dessert: Mixed berry parfait with Greek yogurt.

Day 5:

- Breakfast: Cottage cheese with sliced peaches and a sprinkle of cinnamon.
- Lunch: Whole-grain pasta with tomato, basil, and grilled shrimp.
- Snack: Mixed berries.
- Dinner: Baked chicken breast with quinoa and steamed broccoli.
- Dessert: Sliced mango with a squeeze of lime.

Day 6:

- Breakfast: Whole-grain waffles with fresh raspberries and a dollop of yogurt.
- Lunch: Spinach and arugula salad with grilled salmon and a citrus vinaigrette.
- Snack: Trail mix with almonds, dried cherries, and dark chocolate chips.
- Dinner: Roasted turkey breast with quinoa and roasted Brussels sprouts.
- Dessert: Baked apple with a dash of cinnamon and a dollop of Greek yogurt.

Day 7:

- Breakfast: Greek yogurt parfait with granola, sliced strawberries, and honey.
- Lunch: Chickpea and vegetable curry with brown rice.
- Snack: Sliced cucumber with tzatziki.
- Dinner: Baked trout with a side of quinoa and steamed asparagus.
- Dessert: Sliced kiwi and a piece of dark chocolate.

You are free to modify the ingredients and portion quantities to suit your own dietary requirements and tastes. The Mind Diet ideas can be incorporated into your weekly meals using the meal plans provided here as a starting point. Over time, choosing brain-boosting meals consistently will improve your cognitive health. Enjoy your path to a stronger, healthier mind!

Chapter 8: Lifestyle Tips for a Healthy Mind

To support a healthy and sharp mind, this chapter delves into crucial lifestyle advice and habits that complement the Mind Diet. These lifestyle choices, in addition to nutrition, have a major positive impact on mental health. Following are some important lifestyle suggestions:

Stress Management Techniques

To support a healthy and sharp mind, this chapter delves into crucial lifestyle advice and habits that complement the Mind Diet. These lifestyle choices, in addition to nutrition, have a major positive impact on mental health. Following are some important lifestyle suggestions:

Breathing deeply:

- To relax the nervous system, engage in deep breathing exercises. Take a slow, deep breath in with your nose, hold it for a moment, and then slowly let it out through your lips.
- While concentrating on your breath and letting go of tension, repeat this practice numerous times.

Meditation and Mindfulness:

- You may stay in the moment and lessen the effects of stress by using mindfulness and meditation practices. Set aside some time each day to practice mindfulness.

- This can involve body scans, guided meditation, or just being completely present with your surroundings and feelings.

Regular Exercise:

- Endorphins, which are naturally uplifting chemicals, are released when you exercise. Regular exercise will help you feel better overall and minimize stress.
- Find anything you want to do, whether it's yoga, dancing, cycling, or walking.

Time Management:

- To avoid feeling overwhelmed, prioritize your duties and organize them. Make a to-do list and divide projects into doable steps.
- Utilize time management strategies like the Pomodoro Technique to maintain concentration and productivity.

Healthy Diet:

- Your mood and stress levels may be influenced by a healthy diet. Eat a range of foods that are high in antioxidants, vitamins, and minerals to help your brain function.
- Sugary snacks and excessive caffeine should be avoided as they can cause energy swings and tension.

Social Support:

- Talk to your loved ones about your thoughts and feelings. Social ties offer psychological support and can reduce stress.
- If you need it, don't be afraid to get help from a therapist or counselor.

Sleep Hygiene:

- Make sure you receive enough restorative sleep. Establish a relaxing evening routine and keep a consistent sleep schedule.
- Reduce screen time before bed because the blue light from devices can interfere with sleep cycles.

Relaxation Techniques:

- Investigate relaxing methods like guided imagery, progressive muscle relaxation, and aromatherapy.
- Find the stress-reduction methods that are most effective for you.

Setting Boundaries:

- Get better at saying no to obligations or chores that make you feel overwhelmed. Establish sensible boundaries to safeguard your time and energy.
- Set boundaries with others and put self-care first.

Hobbies and Leisure Activities:

- Take part in interests and pastimes you enjoy. Stress relief can be obtained by engaging in creative or relaxing activities.
- Find what makes you happy, whether it's painting, reading, gardening, or playing music.

Positive Thinking:

- By emphasizing thanksgiving and encouraging affirmations, you can promote a happy outlook.
- Challenge your negative thoughts and recast them from an upbeat standpoint.

Seeking Professional Help:

- Never hesitate to ask a mental health professional for assistance if stress becomes unbearable or chronic.
- Programs for stress management, therapy, or counseling might offer helpful coping mechanisms and emotional support.

Although stress is a normal part of life, it must be carefully managed to safeguard your cognitive health. Try out different variations of these stress-reduction methods to see which one suits you the most, then incorporate it into your daily routine. You can encourage a healthier and more alert mind by lowering stress and fostering mental well-being.

Exercise and Brain Health

Exercise is a potent technique for enhancing cognitive performance and brain health. Exercise has positive effects on both your physical health and the structure and operation of your brain. Here are some ways that physical activity and cognitive health are linked:

1. Improved Blood Flow:

- Your body's blood flow, especially to your brain, improves when you exercise. As a result of improved circulation, the brain receives oxygen and essential nutrients to perform at its best.

2. Neurogenesis:

- Neurogenesis, a process that promotes the growth of new neurons (brain cells), is triggered by physical activity.

Learning and cognitive flexibility are aided by these new neurons.

3. BDNF: A brain-derived neurotrophic factor

- Exercise increases the production of BDNF, a protein that helps neurons develop, maintain, and survive. Increased BDNF levels are linked to better memory and cognitive performance.

4. Neurotransmitter Balance:

- Serotonin and dopamine, neurotransmitters that are important for mood control and cognitive function, are balanced by exercise.
- This harmony might lessen the depressive and anxious sensations that can hinder thinking.

5. Stress Reduction:

- A natural stress reducer is exercise. It lessens the production of stress chemicals like cortisol, which can damage the health of the brain if they are consistently increased.

6. Enhanced Brain Connectivity:

- The connections between various brain regions become stronger with regular activity. This enhanced connection promotes cognitive agility and effective information processing.

7. Cognitive Reserve:

- The idea of cognitive reserve is influenced by physical activity throughout life. The brain can adjust to changes brought on by aging and fend off cognitive loss because of this reserve.

8. Memory and Learning:

- Physical activity throughout life is important for the idea of cognitive reserve. This reserve aids in the brain's ability to adjust to aging-related changes and stave off cognitive decline.

9. Mood Regulation:

- Endorphins, the body's natural mood enhancers, are released when you exercise. Regular exercise helps lessen sadness and anxiety symptoms, which can impair cognitive function.

10. Reduced Inflammation:

- Numerous neurological diseases have been linked to chronic inflammation. Exercise contains anti-inflammatory properties that may lower your risk of developing neurodegenerative illnesses.

11. Better Sleep:

- Better sleep quality can result from regular exercise. For the brain to work properly and to consolidate memories, restorative sleep is crucial.

12. Social Engagement:

- Group classes and team sports are only two examples of workout activities that offer social contact. Social interaction is crucial for cognitive health, especially as you get older.

Aim for a well-rounded fitness regimen that combines aerobic exercises (such as walking, running, and swimming), strength training, flexibility exercises, and balance activities to maximize the advantages of exercise for brain health. Start with a degree of physical exercise appropriate for your level of fitness, then progressively boost the length and intensity.

Recall that consistency is essential. Over time, even little amounts of regular exercise can have a positive effect on the health of your brain. Before beginning a new fitness regimen, speak with a medical expert, especially if you have underlying health issues. You can support a healthier, more alert mind and improve your general quality of life by making physical activity a priority.

Mindful Practices for Mental Clarity

Being completely present and involved in the here and now without passing judgment is a technique known as mindfulness. Developing mindfulness can assist in increasing cognitive function overall, reduce stress, and promote mental clarity. Here are some mindful exercises you can do regularly:

1. Meditation:

- Meditation entails concentrating your attention on a single thing, idea, or breath. Even a few minutes a day of meditation might help with focus and mental clarity.

2. Deep Breathing:

- To clear your mind and soothe your body, try deep breathing techniques. Take a slow, deep breath in with your nose, hold it for a moment, and then let it out through your lips.

3. Mindful Eating:

- Pay special attention to your eating's sensory experience. Enjoy the scents, tastes, and textures of your cuisine.

During meals, stay away from distractions like screens and multitasking.

4. Body Scan:

- To become aware of bodily feelings and tension-filled places in your body, perform a body scan. You can reduce physical tension and increase mental clarity by engaging in this activity.

5. Mindful Walking:

- Take a stroll while paying close attention to your surroundings, the earth beneath your feet, and each step you take. Walking attentively helps you decompress and lowers stress.

6. Gratitude Journaling:

- Keep a thankfulness diary where you can record the things you are grateful for every day. This routine might help you reorient your attention to the good things in life and improve your mental clarity.

7. Mindful Breathing Breaks:

- Throughout the day, schedule brief periods for focused breathing. To calm down, pause and take a few slow, deep breaths.

8. Visualization:

- Use your imagination to place yourself in a calm, focused condition as you engage in positive visualization. Reducing anxiety and increasing mental clarity are two benefits of visualization.

9. Mindful Listening:

- Engage in active listening while you are conversing with others. Without considering your response or any other side issues, give the speaker your undivided attention.

10. Digital Detox:

- Take regular breaks from screens and digital devices. Your mind can get cluttered and less clear if you spend too much time on screens. Spend this time relaxing or engaging in outdoor activities.

11. Progressive Muscle Relaxation:

- Exercises for progressive muscle relaxation might help you relax physically and improve your thinking.

12. Mindful Breathing Before Sleep:

- Before going to bed, practice mindful breathing to clear your thoughts and get better sleep, which is necessary for mental clarity.

13. Mindful Reading:

- Whenever you read a book or an article, give it your full attention. Instead of rushing through text, take your time and enjoy reading.

14. Mindful Cleaning:

- Make routine tasks like cleaning become mindful exercises. Pay attention to the feelings, motions, and sounds made while performing the task.

15. Nature Connection:

- Spend time outdoors and take in your surroundings. A sense of tranquility and mental clarity can be found in nature.

Keep in mind that developing your mindfulness is a skill that takes time. Start with brief sessions and lengthen them gradually as you feel more at ease. These mindful techniques will help you declutter your mind, lessen stress, and improve your cognitive clarity, which will ultimately result in a calmer and more concentrated mind.

Adequate Sleep for Cognitive Wellness

A crucial component of cognitive health is sleep. For several cognitive processes, such as memory consolidation, problem-solving, and emotional control, getting adequate sleep is crucial. Here are some reasons why getting enough sleep is essential for cognitive health and suggestions for enhancing your sleep quality: A Mind-Healthy Sleeping Habit

Why Sleep Matters for Cognitive Wellness:

1. Memory Consolidation: Your brain organizes and consolidates knowledge from the day as you sleep. To learn and retain information, this process is essential.

2. Brain Detoxification: The brain can eliminate toxins and waste particles that accumulate throughout the day as you sleep. This purging procedure promotes ideal brain performance.

3. Emotional Regulation: Getting enough sleep aids with emotion control and lowers the likelihood of mood disorders, anxiety, and depression, all of which hurt cognitive function.

4. Problem-Solving and Creativity: Sleep fosters links between knowledge that at first glance appears to be unconnected, which improves problem-solving skills and increases creativity.

5. Focus and Attention: A good night's sleep increases your ability to focus, pay attention, and concentrate, which makes it easier for you to carry out cognitive tasks.

Tips for Improving Sleep Quality:

1. Consistent Sleep Schedule:

- Even on weekends, go to bed and get up at the same hours every day. Your body's internal clock can be regulated through consistency.

2. Create a Relaxing Bedtime Routine:

- Create a relaxing sleep routine to tell your body it's time to relax. Reading, light stretching, or relaxation techniques are a few possible activities.

3. Comfortable Sleep Environment:

- Make sure the setting where you sleep is relaxing. It is crucial to have a comfy mattress, a pleasant room temperature, and less light and noise.

4. Limit Screen Time Before Bed:

- At least an hour before night, limit your time spent on screens (including TVs, laptops, tablets, and phones). The blue light that screens emit can interfere with your sleep-wake cycle.

5. Mindful Eating and Drinking:

- Avoid consuming large meals, coffee, and alcohol right before bed. These may make it difficult for you to go to sleep and stay asleep.

6. Physical Activity:

- Regular exercise might enhance the quality of sleep. Try to get in at least 30 minutes of moderate exercise most days but stay away from strenuous activity right before night.

7. Manage Stress:

- To relax your body and mind before bed, try stress-reduction exercises like progressive muscle relaxation, deep breathing, or meditation.

8. Limit Naps:

- If you must take a nap during the day, keep it brief (20–30 minutes) and steer clear of afternoon naps because they can disrupt your nocturnal sleep.

9. Watch Your Liquid Intake:

- Reduce fluid intake right before bed to lessen the possibility of waking up to use the restroom.

10. Seek Professional Help:

- If you experience persistent sleep problems or suspect a sleep disorder, check with a healthcare practitioner, or sleep specialist for a full evaluation and treatment options.

Your cognitive health can be significantly improved by making sleep a top priority in your daily schedule. You can promote mental clarity, emotional balance, and general cognitive wellbeing by establishing appropriate sleep habits and a relaxing sleeping environment.

Conclusion

The Mind Diet offers a promising and sustainable route in the pursuit of cognitive wellness and a healthier, sharper mind. By adhering to the dietary approach's guiding principles, you give yourself the power to make conscious food decisions that benefit both your body and mind. The Mind Diet places a strong emphasis on full, nutrient-dense foods that have been connected to enhanced cognitive function and a decreased risk of neurodegenerative disorders.

The Mind Diet, however, is more than simply a list of meals; it's a complete way of life that includes regular exercise, stress reduction, restful sleep, mindfulness exercises, and a dedication to your long-term well-being. These components work together to form an all-encompassing strategy for improving brain health.

Keep in mind that the goal of the Mind Diet is progress, not perfection, as you begin your journey. Your cognitive well-being can be significantly impacted over time by making small, persistent changes to your eating and lifestyle routines. Celebrate your accomplishments, draw lessons from your mistakes, and commit to the long haul on this path.

One of the wisest moves you can do is to invest in the health of your brain, a marvelous organ. You may maximize your cognitive potential and live a more active and satisfying life by feeding your brain with the proper foods, routines, and attitudes.

So, here's to your pursuit of better brain health, to acknowledge your accomplishments, and to the bright, alert mind that awaits you once you adopt the Mind Diet's tenets. May your dedication to cognitive wellness give you energy and well-being for the rest of your life.

Celebrating Your Journey to Improved Brain Health

A wonderful accomplishment is starting a journey to improve your brain health with techniques like the Mind Diet, exercise, mindfulness, and adequate sleep. It's crucial to acknowledge your accomplishments along the way to stay motivated and cultivate a positive outlook. Here are some methods to recognize and honor your progress toward better brain health:

1. Reflect on Achievements:

- Spend some time thinking about the beneficial adjustments you've made to your eating and lifestyle. No matter how minor they may seem, remember to celebrate the victories.

2. Share Your Success:

- Tell your supporters—friends and family—about your journey. Sharing your successes will help you stay more committed to maintaining a healthy brain.

3. Reward Yourself:

- Enjoy prizes that are in line with your path. To celebrate your accomplishments, think about non-food rewards like a spa day, a new book, or a special trip.

4. Keep a Journal:

- Keep a journal to record your travels. Make a list of your objectives, difficulties, and successes. Reading through your journal might serve as a reminder of your successes.

5. Create Positive Habits:

- Keep a journal to record your travels. Make a list of your objectives, difficulties, and successes. Reading through your journal might serve as a reminder of your successes.

6. Share Your Knowledge:

- Tell others about what you've discovered regarding brain health. Helping others on their path by educating them may be satisfying and inspiring.

7. Cultivate Gratitude:

- Embrace thankfulness for the advancements you have encountered. Taking stock of the good improvements in your life might improve your general well-being.

8. Connect with a Community:

- Join a community or group that focuses on nutrition, mindfulness, or brain health. It might be motivating to exchange experiences with others who share your interests.

9. Treat Yourself with Kindness:

- Happy self-compassion day. Be gentle to yourself, especially when things are difficult. Recognize that failures are a necessary part of the trip and can serve as teaching experiences.

10. Acknowledge Progress, Not Perfection:

- Recognize that perfection is not the objective. What matters most are your efforts' advancement and consistency.

11. Set New Goals:

- Continue establishing and achieving fresh objectives for brain health. Your adventure can stay intriguing and new thanks to this continual process.

12. Embrace Mindful Moments:

- Embrace the present moment fully to practice mindfulness. Enjoy the journey itself and the little daily rituals that go along with living a better lifestyle.

13. Celebrate the Journey, Not Just the Destination:

- Keep in mind that your path to better brain health is never over. Celebrate both your destination and your journey's steps.

Long-Term Commitment to the Mind Diet Lifestyle

Remember that there is always more to be done to improve your brain's health. Celebrate your accomplishments along the way and the result. Remember that there is always more to be done to improve your brain's health. Celebrate your accomplishments along the way and the result.

1. Set Realistic Goals:

Remember that there is always more to be done to improve your brain's health. Celebrate your accomplishments along the way and the result. Remember that there is always more to be done to improve your brain's health. Celebrate your accomplishments along the way and the result.

2. Embrace Variety:

Explore a wide range of foods that align with the Mind Diet principles. Incorporate different fruits, vegetables, whole grains, lean proteins, and healthy fats to keep your meals exciting and nutritious.

3. Meal Planning and Preparation:

Make Mind Diet-friendly recipes in advance and plan your meals. Because of this, you won't be tempted to choose less healthy selections when you're stressed for time.

4. Educate Yourself:

Maintain your knowledge of the nutritional advantages of Mind Diet foods. Making thoughtful decisions can be inspired by knowledge of how particular nutrients enhance brain health.

5. Gradual Changes:

It can take some time to adjust to a new nutritional pattern. Make little, steady improvements, and have patience with yourself. Progress, not perfection, is what matters.

6. Mindful Eating:

Enjoy the process of nourishing your body and mind by taking your time with each bite, focusing on the flavors and textures, and practicing mindful eating.

7. Social Support:

Participate in a group of like-minded people who are also on the Mind Diet. Sharing struggles and victories can inspire people and make them feel like they belong.

8. Celebrate Successes:

Celebrate the milestones and accomplishments you've reached on your Mind Diet journey. Recognize the improvements in your health, vitality, and mental acuity.

9. Flexibility:

Be adaptable and flexible. While the Mind Diet offers recommendations, don't be overly strict. Allow yourself to indulge occasionally guilt-free and modify your selections to fit your lifestyle.

10. Continue Learning:

Keep up with the most recent findings in the field of diet and brain health. Learning more can help you stay committed and motivate you to make wise decisions.

11. Listen to Your Body:

Keep track of how your body reacts to various foods. Because everyone has different dietary demands, customize your Mind Diet choices to what is most effective for you.

12. Seek Professional Guidance:

For individualized advice, speak with a qualified dietitian or nutritionist. They can assist you in developing a balanced Mind Diet strategy suited to your requirements.

13. Long-Term Mindset:

Accept the Mind Diet as a way of life rather than a temporary diet. It's a healthy dietary strategy that supports long-term cognitive wellness.

14. Monitor Your Progress:

Regularly evaluate your development and make the required corrections. Keep track of your progress in terms of your general health and cognitive function.

Appendices

Useful Kitchen Tools and Equipment

The proper kitchenware may make meal preparation easier and more fun when following the Mind Diet or any other healthy eating plan. The following is a list of helpful supplies to have in your kitchen:

1. Chef's Knife:

- For chopping, dicing, and slicing fruits and vegetables, a fine chef's knife is required.

2. Cutting Board:

- Pick a sturdy cutting board that can handle your food preparation needs and is easy to clean.

3. Blender or Food Processor:

- These devices are ideal for blending soups, making nutrient-dense sauces, and making smoothies.

4. Vegetable Peeler:

- Use a sharp vegetable peeler to quickly peel and prepare veggies.

5. Salad Spinner:

- Use a sharp vegetable peeler to prepare and peel veggies quickly.

6. Mixing Bowls:

- Mixing bowls of all sizes come in helpful for whisking together ingredients and dressing salads.

7. Measuring Cups and Spoons:

- Keep a set of measuring cups and spoons on hand because precise measurements are essential for baking and cooking.

8. Pots and Pans:

- Invest in a selection of pots and pans, such as a stockpot, saucepan, and non-stick skillet, to prepare a variety of foods.

9. Steamer Basket:

- Using a steamer basket, steam veggies while maintaining their nutrients and flavors.

10. Baking Sheets and Pans:

- For roasting veggies and making nutritious baked items, baking sheets and pans are necessary.

11. Oven Thermometer:

- Make sure the temperature in your oven is perfect for successful baking and roasting.

12. Slow Cooker or Crock-Pot:

- Stews, soups, and one-pot meals can be easily made in slow cookers with little effort.

13. Grater:

- Graters are useful for shredding vegetables, zesting citrus fruits, and grating cheese.

14. Citrus Juicer:

- To use in dishes and drinks, squeeze fresh juice from oranges, limes, and lemons.

15. Food Storage Containers:

- To keep food fresh, store leftovers and meal-ready goods in a variety of airtight containers.

16. Herb and Spice Grinder:

- Freshly ground herbs and spices can enhance the flavor of your food.

17. Kitchen Scale:

- For exact portion control and precise measures when cooking, a kitchen scale is helpful.

18. Can Opener:

- For easy access to canned items like beans and tomatoes, keep a dependable can opener on hand.

19. Colander:

- Using a colander makes it simple to rinse vegetables and drain pasta.

20. Microplate Zester:

- This device is ideal for shredding things like nutmeg, ginger, and garlic very finely.

21. Food Storage Bags:

- For portioning and storing goods in the freezer, use reusable food storage bags.

22. Food Thermometer:

- Use a food thermometer to check the safety and doneness of meat and poultry.

23. Silicone Spatulas and Tongs:

- Silicone non-stick utensils are good for stirring and flipping meals and are kind to cookware.

24. Food Storage Labels:

- Labels on jars and containers will help you keep your refrigerator and pantry organized.

It will be simpler to produce delicious and wholesome meals that are compatible with the Mind Diet if you have access to these kitchen tools and supplies. These tools will be helpful friends in your culinary ambitions as you proceed on your path to better brain health.

Glossary of Mind Diet Ingredients

You may make wise decisions and prepare meals that will enhance your brain function by being aware of the elements that are frequently linked to the Mind Diet. Following is a dictionary of important Mind Diet components:

1. Antioxidants:

Compounds in fruits and vegetables aid in defending the brain against inflammation and oxidative damage. Examples include beta-carotene, vitamin E, and vitamin C.

2. Omega-3 Fatty Acids:

Walnuts and fatty fish like salmon and trout include healthy fats that enhance brain health and lower the risk of cognitive decline.

3. Polyphenols:

Berry, dark chocolate, and green tea are just a few examples of foods that contain plant chemicals with antioxidant qualities. They might aid in enhancing cognitive function.

4. Leafy Greens:

vegetables that are packed with vitamins, minerals, and antioxidants, such as spinach, kale, and Swiss chard.

5. Berries:

Blueberries, strawberries, and raspberries are examples of small, vibrant fruits noted for their high antioxidant content and brain-enhancing qualities.

6. Whole Grains:

Grains that retain all parts of the kernel, including the bran and germ, such as whole wheat, brown rice, quinoa, and oats. They give you fiber and other nutrients.

7. Nuts:

Contains healthy fats, protein, and antioxidants that are good for the brain, such as almonds, walnuts, and cashews.

8. Legumes:

a group of plant-based foods that are high in fiber, protein, different vitamins, and minerals, such as lentils, peas, and beans (such as black beans, and chickpeas).

9. Fatty Fish:

Omega-3 fatty acids, found in fish like salmon, mackerel, and sardines, enhance cognitive function and lower inflammation.

10. Olive Oil:

a monounsaturated fat-rich oil that is good for the heart and a staple of the Mediterranean diet, which is the foundation of the Mind Diet.

11. Avocado:

a fruit that is creamy and rich in nutrients, fiber, and other vitamins and minerals.

12. Poultry:

Protein is available from lean poultry, such as chicken and turkey, without the saturated fat found in red meat.

13. Wine (in Moderation):

Red wine's polyphenol concentration is probably why moderate use of the beverage is linked to some cognitive advantages.

14. Turmeric:

a spice that contains the antioxidant and anti-inflammatory compound curcumin, which may help with brain health.

15. Cinnamon:

a tasty spice that could lower the risk of cognitive decline and manage blood sugar levels.

16. Whole Eggs:

Choline, a vitamin that aids memory and brain function, may be found in eggs.

17. Lean Red Meat (in Moderation):

Lean red meat can be occasionally consumed for its iron and protein content, even if it isn't a focus of the Mind Diet.

18. Whole Milk (in Moderation):

Because they include saturated fat, whole milk, and dairy products should be consumed in moderation.

19. Beans and Lentils:

Legumes that are high in fiber, such as beans and lentils, give you consistent energy and are great sources of plant-based protein.

20. Dark Chocolate (in Moderation):

When consumed in moderation, polyphenols found in dark chocolate with a high cocoa content may help with cognition.

21. Herbs and Spices:

Basil, rosemary, and garlic are flavorful additives that are high in antioxidants and can improve the flavor of Mind Diet recipes.

22. Tomatoes:

Lycopene, a potent antioxidant found in tomatoes, may help to enhance brain function.

Making delicious and brain-boosting choices while adhering to the Mind Diet can be made easier by understanding these essential elements and implementing them into your meals.

Recommended Reading for Further Exploration

The following books provide insightful information if you're keen to learn more about the foundations of the Mind Diet, as well as about brain health, nutrition, and cognitive wellness:

By Maggie Moon, MS, RD, "The Mind Diet: A Scientific Approach to Improving Brain Function and Helping Prevent Alzheimer's and Dementia"

This thorough guide offers a thorough overview of the Mind Diet, its scientific foundation, and helpful advice for applying it to your daily life.

Dean Sherzai, MD, and Ayesha Sherzai, MD, are the authors of "The Alzheimer's Solution: A Breakthrough Program to Prevent and Reverse the Symptoms of Cognitive Decline at Every Age."

This book, which analyzes the connection between lifestyle and brain health and provides tactics to stop and address cognitive decline, was written by eminent neurologists.

Lisa Mosconi, PhD, is the author of "Brain Food: The Surprising Science of Eating for Cognitive Power."

Dr. Mosconi explores the relationship between diet and brain health, describing how certain foods might improve cognitive function and guard against neurodegenerative conditions.

According to Dale Bredesen, MD, "The End of Alzheimer's: The First Program to Prevent and Reverse Cognitive Decline"

Dr. Bredesen offers a novel strategy for halting and reversing cognitive decline through individualized therapies, such as dietary modifications.

Author Valter Longo, Ph., is the author of "The Longevity Diet: Discover the New Science Behind Stem Cell Activation and Regeneration to Slow Aging, Fight Disease, and Optimize Weight."

Dr. Longo investigates the idea of intermittent fasting and its possible advantages for longevity and brain health.

These publications provide a wealth of knowledge, analysis, and useful advice to help you comprehend the Mind Diet, optimize your diet for cognitive wellness, and make wise decisions for a lifestyle that promotes brain health. Happy reading and keep exploring as you work to enhance the health of your brain!

Index

Comprehensive Index

X

- (No Entries)

Y

- (No Entries)

Z

- (No Entries)

This extensive index is intended to make it easy for you to find recipes and interesting subjects in the Mind Diet Cookbook. To obtain the information you need, simply find the appropriate section and page number. Enjoy your path to better brain health through food!

www.ingramcontent.com/pod-product-compliance
Lightning Source LLC
Chambersburg PA
CBHW082221290526
45794CB00009B/3626